VITAMIN A SUPPLEMENTS

A guide to their use in the treatment and prevention of vitamin A deficiency and xerophthalmia

Prepared by a WHO/UNICEF/IVACG Task Force

World Health Organization, Geneva, 1988

The publication of this guide was supported financially by the Government of Italy, through the WHO/UNICEF Joint Nutrition Support Programme.

ISBN 92 4 154236 5

PRINTED IN SWITZERLAND
88/7668-IAM-6000

Contents

Preface

The Thirty-seventh World Health Assembly, in 1984, adopted a resolution requesting the Director-General of the World Health Organization to give all possible support to Member States in the prevention and control of vitamin A deficiency and xerophthalmia and to coordinate the launching and management of action programmes for this purpose with other intergovernmental organizations and appropriate nongovernmental organizations.

In 1985, therefore, WHO proposed a coordinated 10-year plan of action for the prevention and control of vitamin A deficiency and xerophthalmia. The overall strategy includes long-, medium- and short-term measures. Long-term measures are designed to increase the availability and the consumption of foods rich in vitamin A. Medium-term measures include the fortification of food. The administration of high-dose vitamin A supplements to groups at risk constitutes the short-term measure, which can be initiated when urgent and immediate action must be taken.

Programmes for the distribution of vitamin A supplements have expanded steadily over the past three years, so much so that WHO requested the International Vitamin A Consultative Group (IVACG), which provides technical advice on matters related to vitamin A deficiency, to assist in preparing guidelines that could be used by health administrators and programme managers in the development of national or regional programmes for the prevention and control of vitamin A deficiency and xerophthalmia in areas where xerophthalmia constitutes a significant public health problem.

The guidelines presented here have been drawn up by a WHO/UNICEF/IVACG Task Force that considered drafts at meetings held in Brasilia in October 1986 and New York in April 1987 and finalized them in the light of the most recent findings in January 1988 in Washington, DC. They are based on the best scientific evidence available at the present time; nevertheless, it is probable that, with accumulating experience, some changes may need to be introduced in future years.

It is suggested that health administrators and programme managers consider and adapt these guidelines, as they judge appropriate, to their own local conditions and carefully monitor their application. The effects of supplementation programmes on the morbidity and mortality of vitamin-A-deficient persons—children particularly—need further study; national or regional prevention and control programmes offer an excellent opportunity for this.

1. Introduction

Vitamin A supplementation—that is, the periodic administration to vitamin-A-deficient persons of high doses of the vitamin (200 000 IU,[1] or less for special groups)—is effective in controlling vitamin A deficiency and xerophthalmia and in preventing nutritional blindness. To ensure that the vitamin A status of a population becomes and remains adequate requires, of course, more comprehensive, long-term measures that include nutrition education, the fortification with vitamin A of food products such as dried skim milk and sugar, and the production and regular consumption of foods that are naturally rich in vitamin A or provitamin A, such as fish-liver oil and green leafy vegetables. However, high-dose vitamin A supplementation is usually the most effective short-term measure, provided that a sufficient and regular coverage of the population at risk can be achieved. It can be organized relatively quickly at a reasonable cost, and it has an immediate effect in improving the body reserves of vitamin A in the target population. This improvement is important not only for controlling the specific vitamin deficiency, but also for lessening childhood morbidity and mortality due to other causes—diarrhoea and lower respiratory infections, for example. Later, as the more permanent control measures mentioned above take effect, the high-dose supplementation can be phased out.

In areas where vitamin A deficiency and xerophthalmia are known to constitute a significant public health problem (see Annex 2), a sufficient and regular supply of vitamin A preparations should be made available, through the health services system, for distribution at the peripheral level to the local populations at risk. All the personnel at the primary health care level, and community health workers in particular, should be trained in the prevention, recognition, and treatment of xerophthalmia as part of their regular duties.

---

[1] Dosages are expressed in this publication in IU (international units) for the sake of simplicity; see Section 4 for the equivalents in milligrams of retinol.

2. Treatment of xerophthalmia

The treatment schedules given below apply to all stages of active xerophthalmia, including night blindness, conjunctival xerosis, Bitot's spot, corneal xerosis, and keratomalacia. The oral administration of large doses of vitamin A is the recommended method of treatment. The first dose should be given *immediately* xerophthalmia is recognized. Patients with acute corneal lesions should be referred, whenever this is possible, directly to a hospital for treatment of their general condition as well as of their eye disease.

Children under 6 years old

Children over 1 year and under 6 years old

TREAT as shown in Table 1.

Table 1. XEROPHTHALMIA TREATMENT SCHEDULE

for children over 1 year and under 6 years old

Immediately on diagnosis	200 000 IU vitamin A orally (see *Note*)
The following day	200 000 IU vitamin A orally
4 weeks later	200 000 IU vitamin A orally

Note: If there is persistent vomiting or profuse diarrhoea, an intramuscular injection of 100 000 IU of *water-miscible* vitamin A (but *not* an oil-based preparation) may be substituted for the first dose. The use of sterile syringes and needles is, of course, essential.

Children under 1 year old and children of any age who weigh less than 8 kg

TREAT with *half the doses* shown in Table 1.

Notes on the treatment of young children

Children with diarrhoea may absorb rather less of the vitamin A than other children, but if the doses recommended above are used they should still absorb enough for the treatment to be adequate. Xerophthalmic children with severe protein–energy malnutrition need to be carefully monitored because their vitamin A status is unstable and may rapidly worsen, even when they are treated with the doses recommended. Additional doses may then be required for them.

Oil-based preparations are the preferred formulation for oral administration of vitamin A, but water-miscible preparations may be used if the oily solution is not available. If large-dose capsules or concentrated syrup is not available, vitamin A in an equivalent dosage may be given by mouth in other forms, such as fish-liver oil. Oil-based preparations are normally well absorbed by the body when they are administered orally, but they should *never* be injected since oil-based vitamin A is liberated extremely slowly from the injection site. The only preparation suitable for injection, intramuscularly, is water-miscible vitamin A.

Involvement of the cornea in xerophthalmia is a medical emergency. Vitamin A must be administered immediately according to the three-dose schedule in Table 1. In order to treat or reduce the risk of secondary bacterial or viral (measles) infection of the eye, which would compound the damage to the cornea, the topical application of an antibiotic eye ointment, such as tetracycline or chloramphenicol, is recommended. *Ophthalmic ointment containing steroids should never be used in this situation.* To prevent trauma to a cornea already weakened by xerosis or ulceration, the eye should be protected by an eye shield (not occlusive), and it may be necessary to restrain the arm movements of young children by light bandaging.

Children aged 6 years or over, adolescents, and adults (except women of reproductive age)

TREAT with the same dosages as those for children 1 – 6 years old (see Table 1).

Women of reproductive age, pregnant or not

For night blindness or Bitot's spot, TREAT with a daily dose of 10 000 IU of vitamin A orally (1 sugar-coated tablet) for 2 weeks.

When active corneal lesions of xerophthalmia occur in a woman of reproductive age, one has to balance the possible teratogenic or other risk to the fetus (should she be pregnant) of a large dose of vitamin A against the serious consequences for her of vitamin A deficiency if she is not given a large dose. It would appear reasonable, in these exceptional circumstances, to administer the full treatment for corneal xerophthalmia, as described above for young children.

3. Prevention of vitamin A deficiency, xerophthalmia, and nutritional blindness in children

Rationale

Vitamin A (retinol) is a fat-soluble substance that is stored in the human body, principally in the liver, and released as needed into the bloodstream, from which it is drawn for utilization by epithelial cells throughout the body, including those of the eye, and by the photoreceptor cells of the eye. Periodic supplementation with large doses of vitamin A is intended to protect the individual against vitamin A deficiency and its serious consequences over a certain period of time by building up a buffer stock of the vitamin in the liver. Administration of 200 000 IU of vitamin A to a child will give protection for from 3 to 6 months depending on the vitamin A content of the diet and the rate at which the body utilizes it.

Safety

Vitamin A supplementation programmes are known to be effective and safe. When the vitamin A is administered in the doses recommended, there are rarely any adverse effects. Such side-effects as may occur (for instance, headache or vomiting) are minor and transitory and do not require specific treatment.

Disease-targeted distribution

A disease-targeted distribution involves the administration of a high dose of vitamin A to individuals at special risk of developing vitamin A deficiency. Infants and children with infections such as acute or prolonged[1] diarrhoea, acute lower respiratory infections, or severe protein–energy malnutrition who present for treatment at a health

[1] Prolonged diarrhoea means diarrhoea lasting 14 days or more.

centre are the most important groups requiring vitamin A supplementation in any targeted programme. The disease-targeted prevention schedule is given in Table 2.

Table 2. DISEASE-TARGETED PREVENTION SCHEDULE

for preschool children at high risk (e.g., those presenting at a health centre with measles (see *Note 1*), severe protein–energy malnutrition, acute or prolonged diarrhoea, or acute lower respiratory infections)

Children over 1 year and under 6 years old	200 000 IU of vitamin A orally at time of first contact with health worker for each episode of illness (see *Note 2*)
Infants under 1 year old and children of any age who weigh less than 8 kg	100 000 IU of vitamin A orally at time of first contact with health worker for each episode of illness (see *Note 2*)

Note 1: In areas where measles is a particularly severe disease, with a high mortality and a high risk of blindness, as in Africa, it is appropriate to apply the full treatment for xerophthalmia described in Section 2, page 8.

Note 2: This dose should not be given to children who have already received a high-dose vitamin A supplement within the preceding month.

Universal distribution

Universal distribution for prevention in childhood involves the periodic administration of large doses of vitamin A to all children under 6 years old in communities at risk of vitamin A deficiency and a large dose to lactating mothers during the first 2 months after delivery. The prevention schedule is shown in Table 3.

How the doses are spaced in time (from 3 to 6 months apart) will depend upon the amount of vitamin A in the usual diet of the population; it may also be influenced by logistic considerations.

The timing of the distribution of large doses of vitamin A should take account of seasonal factors. Universal-distribution schemes should make vitamin A available to the population before the onset of a season in which there is a special risk of vitamin A deficiency—for instance, seasons when diarrhoea or measles are most frequent or when foods rich in vitamin A are scarce.

Table 3. UNIVERSAL-DISTRIBUTION PREVENTION SCHEDULE

for preschool children and lactating mothers

Children over 1 year and under 6 years old	200 000 IU of vitamin A orally every 3 – 6 months
Infants 6 – 12 months old and any older children who weigh less than 8 kg	100 000 IU of vitamin A orally every 3 – 6 months. Immunization against measles provides a good opportunity to give one of these doses (see *Note*)
Lactating mothers	200 000 IU of vitamin A orally once: at delivery or during the next 2 months. This will raise the concentration of vitamin A in the breast milk and therefore help to protect the breast-fed infant

Note: When infants less than 6 months old are not being breast-fed, supplementation with 50 000 IU of vitamin A before they reach 6 months should be considered.

4. Operational matters

Vitamin A preparations

Although the international unit (IU)—an expression of biological activity rather than of chemical quantity—was officially discontinued as long ago as 1954 for vitamin A (which chemically is retinol), vitamin A preparations are still usually labelled in IU as well as, increasingly, in milligrams (mg) or micrograms (μg) of retinol or its esters. Preparations for vitamin A supplementation may be supplied as retinol palmitate or retinol acetate. Two hundred thousand international units (200 000 IU) are equivalent to 60 mg of retinol, or 110 mg of retinol palmitate, or 69 mg of retinol acetate. In these preparations the vitamin A is usually diluted in a vegetable oil, generally high quality peanut oil, with vitamin E often included as an antioxidant to stabilize the product and to enhance the absorption and storage of vitamin A by the body (e.g., 40 mg (or 40 IU) of vitamin E as *dl*-alpha-tocopherol for 200 000 IU of vitamin A).

The chemical stability and therefore the biological activity of vitamin A are affected by temperature and sunlight; nevertheless, a cold chain is not required in the distribution system. The shelf-life of an oily solution of vitamin A in a properly stored, unopened, opaque container is estimated to be at least 2 years.

Once a container has been opened, however, there is a gradual reduction in the vitamin's biological activity. Partial protection against this is afforded by formulating the oily solution in capsules. Vitamin A, especially in liquid form, should be stored in a dark bottle (or an aluminium container) to shield it from the light. Liquid preparations from properly stored containers should be used within 6 – 8 weeks of opening the container. In general, it is recommended that containers for liquid vitamin A for use in the field or by peripheral health units should be limited in size (e.g., 100 doses) to minimize the loss of potency that may occur once the bottle has been opened. Further information on the stability of vitamin A preparations under various conditions is given in Annex 3.

For the treatment and prevention schedules given in Sections 2 and 3, the following preparations are recommended; they are those contained in the fifth WHO Model List of Essential Drugs (see No. 3 in the Selected Bibliography, page 19):

- Capsules containing 200 000 IU of vitamin A (110 mg of retinol palmitate) in oily solution.

- Oily solution in liquid form for use with dropper or multi-dose dispenser, dispensing a measured dose of vitamin A (e.g., 50 000 IU, or 100 000 IU, or 200 000 IU).
- Sugar-coated tablets, each containing 10 000 IU of vitamin A (5.5 mg of retinol palmitate).
- Ampoules of 2 ml, each containing 100 000 IU of water-miscible vitamin A (55 mg of retinol palmitate) for intramuscular injection.

Logistics

The coverage and continuity of a supplementation programme depend greatly upon supplies being available at the peripheral level when they are needed. At least two factors significantly affect this availability: procurement and distribution.

Procurement

Procurement involves the timely and appropriate purchase of supplies according to the size of the population, its age distribution, and the conditions to be treated. In countries where xerophthalmia is a significant public health problem, for example, vitamin A should be provided for preventive purposes to all preschool children and to mothers after delivery as well as for treating xerophthalmia and other forms of vitamin A deficiency.

To illustrate the type of planning required to determine procurement needs, calculations have been made in the following example for a universal-distribution preventive programme that extends to the treatment of xerophthalmia.

EXAMPLE

(*a*) *Assume* a population of 1000 people with the following characteristics:

- 3% are infants less than 1 year old .... 30 infants
- 3% are children between 1 and 2 years old .... 30 children
- 11% are children over 2 and under 6 years old .... 110 children
- 3% are lactating mothers .... 30 women
- 25% are women of reproductive age (250 women), of whom 4% have night blindness or Bitot's spot .... 10 women
- 5% of the 140 children between 1 and 6 years old have one episode of xerophthalmia per year .... 7 children

(*b*) *Assume* that the following vitamin A preparations are available:

- Capsules containing 200 000 IU of vitamin A in oily solution
- Oily solution in liquid form containing 100 000 IU of vitamin A per 1-ml dose in a multi-dose dispenser
- Sugar-coated tablets containing 10 000 IU of vitamin A

(*c*) *Assume* that infants and children under 2 years old will receive the oily solution from a dispenser and that those 2 years or older will receive a capsule.

(*d*) The *requirements* will be as follows:

Infants:	100 000 IU (1 ml) twice between 6 and 12 months of age for 30 infants	2 ml x 30
Children 1–2 years old:	200 000 IU twice a year for 30 children	4 ml x 30
Children 2–6 years old:	1 capsule of 200 000 IU twice a year for 110 children	220 capsules
Children with xerophthalmia:	3 capsules of 200 000 IU for 7 children	21 capsules
Lactating women:	1 capsule of 200 000 IU for 30 women	30 capsules
Women of reproductive age with night blindness or Bitot's spot:	1 sugar-coated tablet of 10 000 IU per day for 14 days for 10 women	140 tablets

Total per year:	Liquid preparation of vitamin A in dispenser containing 100 000 IU/ml:	(2 ml x 30) + (4 ml x 30) = 180 ml
	Capsules of 200 000 IU:	220 + 21 + 30 = 271 capsules
	Tablets of 10 000 IU:	140 tablets

Cost

Owing to the limited market, very few companies manufacture high-dose vitamin A capsules, and UNICEF is the major global supplier. (In India, however, vitamin A is produced locally and administered to children in the form of a syrup.) The cost per capsule of 200 000 IU of vitamin A (known as retinol high potency in UNICEF essential drugs listings) is less than US$ 0.02 when obtained through UNICEF procurement services. The capsules are available in bottles containing 100 or 500. The cost in other currencies fluctuates according to variations in exchange rates. A handling fee of 4% and a freight charge of 15% by sea are additional.

Distribution

The most important target for vitamin A distribution is the xerophthalmic child. Another vulnerable group that requires immediate attention includes children with infections such as measles, acute or prolonged diarrhoea, and acute lower respiratory infections, or suffering from severe protein–energy malnutrition. Hence any distribution strategy must give priority to the treatment of sick children, whether in a hospital or medical centre or living in their own communities. These, however, represent only a small proportion of all those who would benefit from preventive supplementation with vitamin A.

The timely distribution of a stock of vitamin A preparations from central warehouse to provincial and district stores and thence to field clinics will depend on the existing medical supply system. It will also depend on the perceived need for a supplementation programme, on the resources available, and on the mechanisms at hand for implementing the programme. When universal vitamin A distribution originated, special teams were often formed solely for that purpose, and these were the mainstay of the fledgling programmes of 10 – 15 years ago. Under the influence of new strategies and with the need for economy, however, vitamin A distribution is now being integrated into existing primary health care structures. Although special teams may still be used on occasion, it is generally a routine procedure undertaken within the local health care system.

It is obviously not possible to set out in detail how measures for distributing vitamin A preparations can be incorporated into specific programmes within the health systems of different countries. Nevertheless, programme managers may consider some of the following possibilities, bearing in mind the need to suit measures to the specific situation in each country.

Primary health care/maternal and child health services

Since the adoption in 1978 of the Declaration of Alma-Ata, emphasizing the importance of community outreach in meeting the demands for health care, there has been a move to strengthen and upgrade the primary health care and maternal and child health services. The community health worker is of particular importance here as a critical link between the individual and the health services. The primary health care system being intended to treat the sick and at the same time to monitor the healthy children, it is potentially an effective mechanism into which to integrate vitamin A interventions for both the treatment and the prevention of xerophthalmia and vitamin A deficiency. Some countries have included vitamin A preparations in their essential drugs programmes and thus in the kits of essential drugs supplied to primary health care centres as well as to centres at other levels. This procedure, which facilitates both procurement and distribution, should be adopted in all countries in which xerophthalmia constitutes a significant public health problem.

Programmes for the prevention of blindness

Such programmes exist in an increasing number of developing countries, focusing on action against the major causes of avoidable blindness, which include xerophthalmia. These programmes are usually linked to, or part of, primary health care and include a component of eye care at the community level. This may be utilized for the regular delivery of vitamin A to children and mothers, particularly as they are anyhow often being examined for trachoma in endemic areas or being treated for conjunctivitis or other eye disorders. Furthermore, nutrition education should form part of general education for eye health.

Expanded programmes on immunization

In the many countries in which they have been established, these programmes aim to provide immunization to a target group of young children and to institutionalize the mechanisms for such immunization. They can therefore provide an efficient channel for the distribution of vitamin A to an age group crucial for the control of vitamin A deficiency, though they might miss the 2–3-year-old weanlings and severely malnourished children. It would nevertheless be useful to take advantage of a delivery system that reaches such a large proportion of the critical group.

Diarrhoea control activities

The child who suffers from acute or prolonged diarrhoea also runs a special risk of vitamin A deficiency. Oral rehydration therapy at a health centre provides a mechanism by which children who may need supplemental vitamin A can be identified and given it.

Other channels

Channels outside the usual scope of the health care system have also been used for vitamin A supplementation. Among these are the school system, agricultural extension schemes, mothers' groups, and nongovernmental organizations and voluntary agencies. Indeed, several nongovernmental organizations have been, and still are, actively supporting vitamin A supplementation schemes as part of their contribution to development work.

Training

In order to ensure the maximum coverage of vulnerable population groups, the entire health system must be involved and its personnel must be proficient in recognizing the signs and symptoms of vitamin A deficiency and in its treatment and prevention. The medical staff needs to be able to recognize and treat the condition and to deal with patients referred to them from other points in the system. The community health workers need instruction in identification, prevention, treatment, and referral. The specific schedules for treatment and prevention must be known to the staff at all levels of the health system as well as to any other persons involved in the work for the control of vitamin A deficiency.

The most efficient way to ensure the regular provision of the required training is to integrate a vitamin A component into the existing curricula for health workers at all levels. Teaching materials have been developed by WHO[1] and by other organizations such as Helen Keller International Incorporated,[2] which can easily be inserted into formal training sessions.

Monitoring and evaluation

Monitoring

Monitoring in this context is essentially a means of determining whether or not vitamin A is being appropriately delivered, where, and to whom. It is a useful supervisory tool for programme management and invaluable for indicating problems of supply and logistics as they occur. For this purpose it is recommended to include a record of vitamin A administration in existing record forms, such as growth charts, mothers' cards, and health centre records. This is particularly important if several channels are being used for the delivery of vitamin A as it helps to avoid duplication while ensuring safety and full coverage.

Evaluation

A simple type of evaluation is to measure whether or not a supplementation programme has reached its goals in terms of vitamin A distribution. It initially involves identifying a target population and the intended level of coverage, then following through to determine whether the vitamin A is reaching that population at the intended level. Existing record systems can be used, and surveillance teams can gather additional information to supplement the data from those records. Evaluation of programme impact (i.e., whether or not the incidence and prevalence of vitamin A deficiency have declined since the start of a programme's activities) is more complex; it requires greater resources but is invaluable in motivating politicians, health administrators, and the public to support the programme. It will also help to determine whether further operational research is necessary to adjust the distribution strategy to local conditions; this is especially true for disease-targeted programmes, which deal with a spectrum of pathological conditions whose frequency and severity vary from place to place.

---

1 For information write to: Nutrition, Division of Family Health, World Health Organization, 1211 Geneva 27, Switzerland.

2 For information write to: Helen Keller International Incorporated, 15 West 16th Street, New York, NY 10011, USA.

Selected bibliography

Publications of the World Health Organization[1]

1. WHO Technical Report Series, No. 590, 1976 (*Vitamin A deficiency and xerophthalmia:* report of a Joint WHO/USAID Meeting).
2. WHO Technical Report Series, No. 672, 1982 (*Control of vitamin A deficiency and xerophthalmia:* report of a Joint WHO/UNICEF/USAID/Helen Keller International/IVACG Meeting).
3. WHO Technical Report Series, No. 770, 1988 (*The use of essential drugs:* third report of the WHO Expert Committee).
4. Sommer, A. *Field guide to the detection and control of xerophthalmia*, 2nd ed. Geneva, World Health Organization, 1982.
5. *Weekly epidemiological record*, **62** (19): 133-134 (1987) (Joint WHO/UNICEF statement on vitamin A for measles).
6. World Health Organization. *Prevention and control of vitamin A deficiency, xerophthalmia and nutritional blindness: proposal for a ten-year programme of support to countries.* Unpublished document NUT/84.5 Rev. 1 (Available upon request from Nutrition, Division of Family Health, WHO, 1211 Geneva 27, Switzerland).

Publications of the United Nations Administrative Committee on Coordination/Sub-Committee on Nutrition[2]

7. West, K.W. & Sommer, A. *Delivery of oral doses of vitamin A to prevent vitamin A deficiency and nutritional blindness.* 1987 (Nutrition Policy Discussion Paper No. 2).

Publications of the United Nations Children's Fund[3]

8. *Essential drugs: Price list.* Copenhagen, UNICEF (published twice yearly).
9. Eastman, S.J. *Vitamin A deficiency and xerophthalmia. Recent findings and some programme implications.* New York, UNICEF, 1987.

Publications of the International Vitamin A Consultative Group[4]

10. International Vitamin A Consultative Group. *Guidelines for the eradication of vitamin A deficiency and xerophthalmia.* Washington, DC, IVACG, 1977.
11. De Luca, L.M. et al. *Recent advances in the metabolism and function of vitamin A and their relationship to applied nutrition.* Washington, DC, IVACG, 1979.

[1] References 1-5 are available from Distribution and Sales, World Health Organization, 1211 Geneva 27, Switzerland.

[2] Available from ACC/SCN, c/o World Health Organization, 1211 Geneva 27, Switzerland.

[3] Available from UNICEF, UNICEF House, 3 United Nations Plaza, New York, NY 10017, USA.

[4] Available from International Life Sciences Institute – Nutrition Foundation, 1126 Sixteenth Street NW, Washington, DC 20036, USA.

12. BAUERNFEIND, J.C. *The safe use of vitamin A*. Washington, DC, IVACG, 1980.
13. MCLAREN, D.S. ET AL. *The symptoms and signs of vitamin A deficiency and their relationship to applied nutrition*. Washington, DC, IVACG, 1981.
14. INTERNATIONAL VITAMIN A CONSULTATIVE GROUP. *Biochemical methodology for the assessment of vitamin A status*. Washington, DC, IVACG, 1982.
15. WEST, K.P. & SOMMER, A. *Periodic large oral doses of vitamin A for the prevention of vitamin A deficiency and xerophthalmia: a summary of experiences*. Washington, DC, IVACG, 1984.
16. UNDERWOOD, B.A. *The safe use of vitamin A by women during the reproductive years*. Washington, DC, IVACG, 1986.

Publications from the International Center for Epidemiologic and Preventive Ophthalmology[1]

17. SOMMER, A. ET AL. Oral versus intramuscular vitamin A in the treatment of xerophthalmia. *Lancet*, **1**: 557-559 (1980).
18. SOMMER, A. *Nutritional blindness: xerophthalmia and keratomalacia*. New York, Oxford University Press, 1982.
19. SOMMER, A. ET AL. Increased mortality in children with mild vitamin A deficiency. *Lancet*, **2**: 585-588 (1983).
20. SOMMER, A. ET AL. Increased risk of respiratory disease and diarrhoea in children with pre-existing mild vitamin A deficiency. *American journal of clinical nutrition*, **40**: 1090-1095 (1984).
21. SOMMER A. ET AL. Impact of vitamin A supplementation on childhood mortality. *Lancet*, **1**: 1169-1173 (1986).

[1] Address: Dana Center, Wilmer Institute, Johns Hopkins Hospital, 600 North Wolfe Street, Baltimore, MD 21205, USA.

Annex 1

Participants in the WHO/UNICEF/IVACG Task Force

Dr C.O. Chichester, International Vitamin A Consultative Group, Washington, DC, USA

Dr N. Cohen, Geneva, Switzerland (WHO Consultant)

Dr F. Davidson, Office of Nutrition, United States Agency for International Development, Washington, DC, USA

Dr E.M. DeMaeyer, Geneva, Switzerland (WHO Consultant) (*Chairman*)

Ms S.J. Eastman, Helen Keller International Incorporated, New York, NY, USA

Dr J.P. Greaves, United Nations Children's Fund, New York, NY, USA

Dr R. Leavell, Helen Keller International Incorporated, New York, NY, USA

Dr D.S. McLaren, University of Edinburgh, Edinburgh, Scotland

Dr L.H. Pacheco-Santos, Federal University of Paraíba João Pessoa, Paraíba, Brazil

Dr F. Solon, Nutrition Centre of the Philippines, Manila, Philippines

Dr A. Sommer, International Center for Epidemiologic and Preventive Ophthalmology, Wilmer Institute, Johns Hopkins Hospital, Baltimore, MD, USA

Dr L.J. Teply, International Vitamin A Consultative Group, Washington, DC, USA

Dr B.A. Underwood, National Eye Institute, National Institutes of Health, Bethesda, MD, USA

Dr K.P. West, Jr, International Center for Epidemiologic and Preventive Ophthalmology, Wilmer Institute, Johns Hopkins Hospital, Baltimore, MD, USA

Annex 2

Countries categorized by degree of public health significance of vitamin A deficiency, xerophthalmia, and nutritional blindness

(From information available to WHO in January 1988)

WHO Region	Category 1[a]	Category 2[b]	Category 3[c]
Africa	Benin Burkina Faso Chad Ethiopia Ghana Malawi Mali Mauritania Niger Nigeria United Republic of Tanzania Zambia	Angola Kenya Mozambique Uganda Rwanda Burundi	Algeria Botswana Lesotho Madagascar Senegal Zaire Zimbabwe
Americas	Brazil Haiti	El Salvador Guatemala Honduras	Bolivia Ecuador Jamaica Mexico Peru
South-East Asia	Bangladesh India Indonesia Nepal Sri Lanka	Burma Bhutan	Thailand
Europe			Turkey

[a] Category 1: Significant public health problem in part or whole of country.

[b] Category 2: Insufficient information but high probability of significant public health problem in part or whole of country.

[c] Category 3: Sporadic cases but prevalence not such that it constitutes a significant public health problem.

WHO Region	Category 1	Category 2	Category 3
Eastern Mediterranean	Sudan	Afghanistan Pakistan	Egypt Iran, Islamic Republic of Iraq Jordan Morocco Oman Somalia Syrian Arab Republic Yemen
Western Pacific	Philippines Viet Nam	Democratic Kampuchea Lao People's Democratic Republic	China Fiji Malaysia

Annex 3

Data on the stability of commonly supplied vitamin A preparations

Vitamin A (as retinol palmitate) in oily solution, 10^6 IU/g; stabilized with *dl-α*-tocopherol

Storage conditions: 5 °C, room temperature, 35 °C; unopened container.

Storage temperature	Retinol retention after:		
	6 months	12 months	24 months
5 °C	99 %	98 %	97 %
Room temperature	99 %	95 %	92 %
35 °C	97 %	92 %	76 %

Source: Hoffmann La Roche, Basle, Switzerland.

Vitamin A (as retinol palmitate) in edible oil contained in soft gelatine capsules

Storage conditions: 23 °C; closed containers.

Capsulation run	Initial retinol content (IU/capsule)	Retinol retention (after indicated storage time)
1	214 000	99 % (20 months)
2	209 000	99 % (29 months)
3	214 000	97 % (31 months)

Source: Hoffmann La Roche, Nutley, NJ, USA.

WHO publications may be obtained, direct or through booksellers, from:

ALGERIA: Entreprise nationale du Livre (ENAL), 3 bd Zirout Youcef, ALGIERS

ARGENTINA: Carlos Hirsch SRL, Florida 165, Galerías Güemes, Escritorio 453/465, BUENOS AIRES

AUSTRALIA: Hunter Publications, 58A Gipps Street, COLLINGWOOD, VIC 3066

AUSTRIA: Gerold & Co., Graben 31, 1011 VIENNA I

BAHRAIN: United Schools International, Arab Region Office, P.O. Box 726, BAHRAIN

BANGLADESH: The WHO Representative, G.P.O. Box 250, DHAKA 5

BELGIUM: *For books:* Office International de Librairie s.a., avenue Marnix 30, 1050 BRUSSELS. *For periodicals and subscriptions:* Office International des Périodiques, avenue Louise 485, 1050 BRUSSELS

BHUTAN: *see* India, WHO Regional Office

BOTSWANA: Botsalo Books (Pty) Ltd., P.O. Box 1532, GABORONE

BRAZIL: Centro Latinoamericano de Informação em Ciencias de Saúde (BIREME), Organização Panamericana de Saúde, Sector de Publicações, C.P. 20381 - Rua Botucatu 862, 04023 SÃO PAULO, SP

BURMA: *see* India, WHO Regional Office

CAMEROON: Cameroon Book Centre, P.O. Box 123, South West Province, VICTORIA

CANADA: Canadian Public Health Association, 1335 Carling Avenue, Suite 210, OTTAWA, Ont. K1Z 8N8. (Tel: (613) 725–3769. Télex: 21–053–3841)

CHINA: China National Publications Import & Export Corporation, P.O. Box 88, BEIJING (PEKING)

DEMOCRATIC PEOPLE'S REPUBLIC OF KOREA: *see* India, WHO Regional Office

DENMARK: Munksgaard Export and Subscription Service, Nørre Søgade 35, 1370 COPENHAGEN K (Tel: +45 1 12 85 70)

FIJI: The WHO Representative, P.O. Box 113, SUVA

FINLAND: Akateeminen Kirjakauppa, Keskuskatu 2, 00101 HELSINKI 10

FRANCE: Arnette, 2, rue Casimir-Delavigne, 75006 PARIS

GERMAN DEMOCRATIC REPUBLIC: Buchhaus Leipzig, Postfach 140, 701 LEIPZIG

GERMANY, FEDERAL REPUBLIC OF: Govi-Verlag GmbH, Ginnheimerstrasse 20, Postfach 5360, 6236 ESCHBORN — Buchhandlung Alexander Horn, Kirchgasse 22, Postfach 3340, 6200 WIESBADEN

GREECE: G. C. Eleftheroudakis S.A., Librairie internationale, rue Nikis 4, 105-63 ATHENS

HONG KONG: Hong Kong Government Information Services, Publication (Sales) Office, Information Services Department, No. 1, Battery Path, Central, HONG KONG

HUNGARY: Kultura, P.O.B. 149, BUDAPEST 62

INDIA: WHO Regional Office for South-East Asia, World Health House, Indraprastha Estate, Mahatma Gandhi Road, NEW DELHI 110002

IRAN (ISLAMIC REPUBLIC OF): Iran University Press, 85 Park Avenue, P.O. Box 54/551, TEHERAN

IRELAND: TDC Publishers, 12 North Frederick Street, DUBLIN 1 (Tel: 744835–749677)

ICELAND: Snaebjorn Jonsson & Co., Hafnarstraeti 9, P.O. Box 1131, IS-101 REYKJAVIK

ISRAEL: Heiliger & Co., 3 Nathan Strauss Street, JERUSALEM 94227

ITALY: Edizioni Minerva Medica, Corso Bramante 83–85, 10126 TURIN; Via Lamarmora 3, 20100 MILAN; Via Spallanzani 9, 00161 ROME

JAPAN: Maruzen Co. Ltd, P.O. Box 5050, TOKYO International, 100–31

JORDAN: Jordan Book Centre Co. Ltd., University Street, P.O. Box 301 (Al-Jubeiha), AMMAN

KENYA: Text Book Centre Ltd, P.O. Box 47540, NAIROBI

KUWAIT: The Kuwait Bookshops Co. Ltd, Thunayan Al-Ghanem Bldg, P.O. Box 2942, KUWAIT

LAO PEOPLE'S DEMOCRATIC REPUBLIC: The WHO Programme Coordinator, P.O. Box 343, VIENTIANE

LUXEMBOURG: Librairie du Centre, 49 bd Royal, LUXEMBOURG

MALAYSIA: The WHO Representative, Room 1004, 10th Floor, Wisma Lim Foo Yong (formerly Fitzpatrick's Building), Jalan Raja Chulan, KUALA LUMPUR 05–10; P.O. Box 2550, KUALA LUMPUR 01–02 — Parry's Book Center, 124–1 Jalan Tun Sambanthan, P.O. Box 10960, KUALA LUMPUR

MALDIVES: *see* India, WHO Regional Office

MEXICO: Librería Interacademica S.A., av. Sonora 206, 06100-MÉXICO, D.F.

MONGOLIA: *see* India, WHO Regional Office

MOROCCO: Editions La Porte, 281 avenue Mohammed V, RABAT

NEPAL: *see* India, WHO Regional Office

NETHERLANDS: Medical Books Europe BV, Noorderwal 38, 7241 BL LOCHEM

NEW ZEALAND: New Zealand Government Printing Office, Publishing Administration, Private Bag, WELLINGTON; Walter Street, WELLINGTON; World Trade Building, Cubacade, Cuba Street, WELLINGTON. *Government Bookshops at:* Hannaford Burton Building, Rutland Street, Private Bag, AUCKLAND; 159 Hereford Street, Private Bag, CHRISTCHURCH; Alexandra Street, P.O. Box 857, HAMILTON; T & G Building, Princes Street, P.O. Box 1104, DUNEDIN — R. Hill & Son, Ltd, Ideal House, Cnr Gillies Avenue & Eden St., Newmarket, AUCKLAND 1

NORWAY: Tanum — Karl Johan A.S., P.O. Box 1177, Sentrum, N-0107 OSLO 1

PAKISTAN: Mirza Book Agency, 65 Shahrah–E–Quaid–E–Azam, P.O. Box 729, LAHORE 3

PAPUA NEW GUINEA: The WHO Representative, P.O. Box 646, KONEDOBU

PHILIPPINES: World Health Organization, Regional Office for the Western Pacific, P.O. Box 2932, MANILA; National Book Store Inc., 701 Rizal Avenue, P.O. Box 1934, MANILA

PORTUGAL: Livraria Rodrigues, 186 Rua da Ouro, LISBON 2

REPUBLIC OF KOREA: The WHO Representative, Central P.O. Box 540, SEOUL

SAUDI ARABIA: World of Knowledge for Publishing and Distribution, P.O. Box 576, JEDDAH

SINGAPORE: The WHO Representative, 144 Moulmein Road, SINGAPORE 1130; Newton P.O. Box 31, SINGAPORE 9122

SOUTH AFRICA: *Contact major book stores*

SPAIN: Comercial Atheneum S.A., Consejo de Ciento 130–136, 08015 BARCELONA; General Moscardó 29, MADRID 20 — Librería Díaz de Santos, P.O. Box 6050, 28006 MADRID; Balmes 417 y 419, 08022 BARCELONA

SRI LANKA: *see* India, WHO Regional Office

SWEDEN: *For books:* Aktiebolaget C.E. Fritzes Kungl. Hovbokhandel, Regeringsgatan 12, 103 27 STOCKHOLM. *For periodicals:* Wennergren-Williams AB, Box 30004, 104 25 STOCKHOLM

SWITZERLAND: Medizinischer Verlag Hans Huber, Länggassstrasse 76, 3012 BERN 9

THAILAND: *see* India, WHO Regional Office

UNITED KINGDOM: H.M. Stationery Office: 49 High Holborn, LONDON WCIV 6HB; 71 Lothian Road, EDINBURGH EH3 9AZ; 80 Chichester Street, BELFAST BT1 4JY; Brazennose Street, MANCHESTER M6O 8AS; 258 Broad Street, BIRMINGHAM B1 2HE; Southey House, Wine Street, BRISTOL BS1 2BQ. *All mail orders should be sent to:* HMSO Publications Centre, 51 Nine Elms Lane, LONDON SW8 5DR

UNITED STATES OF AMERICA: *Copies of individual publications (not subscriptions):* WHO Publications Center USA, 49 Sheridan Avenue, ALBANY, NY 12210. *Subscription orders and correspondence concerning subscriptions should be addressed to the* World Health Organization, Distribution and Sales, 1211 GENEVA 27, Switzerland. *Publications are also available from the* United Nations Bookshop, NEW YORK, NY 10017 *(retail only)*

USSR: *For readers in the USSR requiring Russian editions:* Komsomolskij prospekt 18, Medicinskaja Kniga, MOSCOW — *For readers outside the USSR requiring Russian editions:* Kuzneckij most 18, Meždunarodnaja Kniga, MOSCOW G-200

VENEZUELA: Librería Médica Paris, Apartado 60.681, CARACAS 106

YUGOSLAVIA: Jugoslovenska Knjiga, Terazije 27/II, 11000 BELGRADE

ZIMBABWE: Textbook Sales (PVT) Ltd, 1 Norwich Union Centre, MUTARE

Special terms for developing countries are obtainable on application to the WHO Representatives or WHO Regional Offices listed above or to the World Health Organization, Distribution and Sales Service, 1211 Geneva 27, Switzerland. Orders from countries where sales agents have not yet been appointed may also be sent to the Geneva address, but must be paid for in pounds sterling, US dollars, or Swiss francs. Unesco book coupons may also be used.

Prices are subject to change without notice. C/1/88